HOW TO DETOX FOR

GREAT HEALTH

How To Detox For Great Health

Body Detox And Colon
Cleansing For Health And A
Quick Weight Loss

Debra Richards

TABLE OF CONTENT

Body Detox

Body detoxification is something very popular in recent years. This is especially evident in popular celebrities' culture. Everyone seems to be on this detox trend nowadays.

This is very popular for a reason. It is very healthy for your body. You may have wondered about it and asked about how it would help you. As a form of colon cleansing, body detoxification would conjure unpleasant images in your mind.

However, once you understand body detox and the science behind it, you will start to understand the benefits of it.

The purpose of detoxification is to slowly clean out your digestive system. This is done by drinking a solution made to clean your intestines and to boost your organs in your digestive system.

This is merely done by simply drinking the right drinks, doing the right things and then going to a bathroom. As simple as that. This helps your digestive system get healthy. This would help your digestive system work well. If it is unhealthy, your whole body would suffer in the long run. A strong digestive system would help you have a healthier body.

It doesn't matter if you are a person who doesn't smoke or drink. But if your digestive system is filled with toxins, you would still be unhealthy. From the food you eat to the air of breath, there are toxins everywhere. Such toxins would linger around your body and would affect your digestive system. As said before, your digestive system is extremely important to maintaining your good health.

Simply put, our digestive system is made up of several organs. This includes your liver, kidneys, intestines and pancreas. Each of them have their important roles. When you eat, the food enters the digestive system through the stomach and is passed for processing through your digestive tract.

Certain foods and drinks, when taken, would make the kidneys and pancreas having to work overtime to process them. Every single organ in your digestive system has a very job to ensure that your body is healthy. As the food and drinks are processed by your system, it would be eliminated by waste.

However, this doesn't mean that it work like that always. Certain times, the food you eat would end up stuck in your intestines. For some people, this is so serious that some elements are in their intestines for 10 years.

Some of these are toxins and getting rid of them is extremely difficult. Certain foods like simple carbohydrates are very hard for your kidneys to process. Your organs would need to work overtime in order to make it work.

Another important factor that affects the toxins in your body is the air that your breath. There are a lot of toxins in the air. For example, this may include the second-hand smoke that your breathe which is absorbed into your bloodstream. This would invariably affect your digestive system.

Your body would also absorb toxins when you take a bath or shower. This is because your skin could absorb those chemicals that are in shampoo and soap. This itself would affect the amount of toxins in your body as well.

You can't live your life toxin free. You may try hard to live such a life, but it is inevitable that you pick up certain germs from the air.

Therein lies the power of body detoxification. Body detoxification would help your body clean itself of all the toxins or foods that are stuck in your digestive system. It isn't only good for health, but would help you lose weight as well. Just by performing body detox, I find that many people could easily lose a few pounds.

When you take body detoxification fluid, it is pretty much similar to barium enema. The only difference is that you don't have to drink so much and it tastes so much better. Barium enema would clear your intestines and is normally given to those who would have tests done on their digestive organs.

This fluid would eliminate the waste from your body and makes you feel lighter. It wouldn't only get rid of toxins, but would get rid of other waste which lingers around your intestines.

To become healthier, the first step is to drink body detoxification formula. However, you cannot just stop there. You would need to change your lifestyle and create empowering habits.

You should look to eat right, exercise regularly and remove your unhealthy lifestyle. Body detoxification is a manner to enhance your health, help you lose weight and ensure that you have a digestive system which is healthy.

Done well, body detoxification would fill your body with the right nutrients that you lack previously. This would ensure that you are healthier over the long term.

This book would give you a step by step guide towards understanding the process of body detoxification and perform it from the comfort of your home. It would cover about creating a healthy lifestyle.

We would cover all the aspects about body detoxification, deciding if you should perform it and the steps to make your own body detoxification treatments from home.

At the end of this book, you would have the knowledge needed regardless of your intention. From being healthy, losing weight or improving your digestive system; this book would guide you.

Who Needs Body Detox

Anyone can get the great benefits from the use of body detox. However, how you perform it very much depend on the lifestyle that you live as well as your intention of body detox. If you are someone with an unhealthy lifestyle, a body detox would probably help you even more.

If you are already healthy and just want to maintain a good digestive health, you could perform body detox less often than someone who isn't healthy. Regardless of where you are, everybody needs a good body detox to improve our digestive system.

Keep Digestive System Healthy

To ensure that you are healthy, the health of your digestive system is perhaps the most important. According to cancer research, colon cancer is the third cancer killer in the United States of America.

Colon cancer, the cancer of the small intestine is due to polyps in your colon. Body detox helps you get rid of these wastes in your body and ensures that your colon is clean.

Not only that, body detox also helps to feed your organs with the right nutrients. Body detox formulas have vitamins, herbs and minerals that would assist your body in cleaning your digestive system and would also feed nutrients into your organs.

That is the reason why many people feel extremely refreshed after a body detox. Your digestive system is healthy and you will feel good.

When you consume natural body detox supplements, your body is being fed nutrients that would assist not just your digestive system, but your entire body. Your digestive organs would send nutrients to your entire body, brain and other vital organs. Body detox helps your entire body.

People Who Want To Lose Weight

Body detox is a great method if you want to lose weight. This helps your body get rid of the waste and you would feel much lighter from here. Those who are looking for a method of losing weight would opt for a good body detox. It is very healthy for weight loss.

Many of us feel bloated and retain a great deal of our weight because we store the waste in our digestive system. Body detox helps you lose the waste and you would feel lighter quickly. However, you need to be aware that body detox isn't a laxative and it is a more natural way of eliminating waste from your system. These would lead to greater weight loss.

Get Rid Of Toxins

In Hollywood, many popular celebrities are commonly using body detox in order to get rid of the toxins that are in their body. With a proper body cleanse system; you are able to remove the toxins from your body.

This works well towards making sure that your body is clean and is free from the poisons that are consumed by the body.

For those people with unhealthy lifestyle, a body detox is a great way to stay healthier and remove toxins from your body. This is especially helpful for those people who are smokers, drinkers and those with unhealthy diet.

Although body detox isn't sufficient, it helps. In order to make an overall change in your health, the important thing to do is to change your lifestyle habits.

Body detox just helps remove the toxins that are in your body. It would rid your body of the toxins that you come into contact daily. Remember, body detox isn't just good for your digestive system but your overall health.

Pass Drug Testing

It is very common for those people to use body detox to clean their body to remove remnants of illegal substances from their body. This is because they are about to be drug-tested for a certain jobs. Although it may not completely help them pass the drug blood test, it could assist you in passing your urine test for tobacco or drugs.

Although it isn't recommended that you use body detox to pass drug tests, it would help you if you happen to make a bad decision in the past and want to repent. Everyone makes mistakes, and consuming drugs may be one of them. A sudden lapse of judgment may result in this and using body detox to rid your body of toxins would help you pass the test.

Taking Supplements

For this purposes, there are multiple products that are on the market. Most of them aren't just to detox your body from toxins, but to ensure that you would maintain your good health.

Different product has different purposes depending on what you want to use it for. From losing weight to maintaining good health, you need to check on the purpose of the product beforehand.

However, you may even create your own solutions from the comfort of your home. Using natural ingredients, home remedies could be used to detox without the need of supplements. In the later chapters of this book, you would learn how to use those formulas and use it easily.

While body detox is easily performed from the comfort of your home, this shouldn't be a substitute for common sense. While body detox helps you remove toxins, lose weights or pass drug tests; you need to realize that the most important thing to staying healthy is to avoid toxins, drugs and have positive lifestyle habits.

Using Body Detox For Weight Loss

It is very difficult to lose weight. It is even more so if you want to do it fast. Among the main purposes of a body detox is because to help you lose weight quick. Besides losing weight, you would also improve your body with the right nutrients you need while losing weight at the same time.

Although there are several pills for weight loss in the market, nothing beats losing weight through body detox. And for this to happen, the main thing you need to use is water. Use herbal supplements with vitamins, together with water to ensure that you lose weight. Pre-made solutions could also be used. You could purchase them online or through health stores as a weight loss remedy over the long term.

Perhaps it sounds very simple, but drinking a lot of water is one of the best and safest ways to permanent weight loss. Water fills you us and help you expel the excess water in your body.

It is highly recommended to drink at least eight glasses of water in a day whether you are on a body detox or not. However, it is even more important when you want to lose weight. However, water isn't sufficient for weight loss.

You also need to make sure that your body is filled with the right nutrients. When you are trying to lose weight, many would look to skip meals and vitamins are therefore very important.

You also need to ensure that your digestive tract is clean and to make sure that the waste in your body is disposed from your body. Taking body detoxification supplements would also assist your body with the vitamins required while you are looking to lose weight.

But, nothing beats the safety that comes from a body detox. Weight loss pills that often contain ingredients may be unhealthy as well. You can make your own body detox solution with mixes water with other ingredients that would help clean your system. Besides such mixtures, you could even purchase other commercial products for this purpose.

Body detox systems is a much safer alternative than using diet drinks that act as laxatives and contain unhealthy chemicals. When looking for a solution towards detoxifying your body, it is highly recommended to seek a system that incorporates all the natural ingredients.

It is much better to consume a system filled with natural ingredients that one which is filled with chemicals because it would not only assist you with weight loss but promote a healthier well-being.

When one thinks of weight loss through detox, perhaps the most important natural herb is **green tea**. The power of green tea lies in its ability to act like a diuretic to quicken the weight loss process.

To get the best out of it, you should look to drink it plain, without sugar. In fact, I have known people who drink green tea all day long instead of water. This is especially common in Japan. If you dislike the taste of green tea, you could even buy its tablet alternative.

Another great herb is cranberry. When you take cranberries, it is recommended to take it in its tablet form as drinks that you purchase from your grocery store are heavily loaded with sugar. When you consume cranberry, you also help your body clear the urinary tract.

Another very common method for detox to lose weight is to create your own solutions. Many of them are marketed as colon cleansers. It is very important that you focus on cleaning your colons if you want to ensure that you lose weight as quick as you can.

Such methods would clean the waste in your intestines to speed up the weight loss process.

When on such detox to lose weight, water is also very important because it assist the detox process. Dieting alone is insufficient if you don't consume the right liquids.

However, you need to remember that a body detox isn't a magic formula that works instantly. If done wrongly, you may create detrimental effects. As much as you want to lose weight, you still need to practice some common sense. Do more exercises and consume a good amount of calories.

Used well, body detoxification could be an asset towards your goal of losing weight and improving your physical well-being.

Using Body Detox For Simply Detoxing

This is perhaps the main reason why people perform a body detox. From the mere comfort of your home, you are able to perform it and maintain a healthier body.

To perform it, there are several different products in the market which you can use. Like said in the previous chapter, different products have different purposes. You need to be sure of the right one to take.

Normally, body detox is done with a drinkable solution. There are teas and tablets to take as well. Home kits for body detox would often consist of tablets and teas together with water solutions. It is normally recommended to buy such kits than to buy individual products as it is not only cheaper but more effective as well.

Depending on your lifestyle, you should look to detox your body once in a while. If you are someone who takes in a lot of toxins, you should use it once a week. You could simply just mix those solutions with water and then drink it. A majority of the solutions have very nice taste and works almost immediately upon drinking them.

You also need to drink a lot of water to ensure that the process goes on smoothly. Most packaging would also include an instruction on how much water you should drink after taking those solutions. Follow those instructions as the water would help the detox product flush through your system and quicken the detox process.

A body detox would also help you get rid of ailments in your body. If you have stress, cold or other physical ailment; you would be surprised with how a simply body detox would help you feel better.

Ideally speaking, a home kit is a great tool when looking to body cleanse for health purposes. It is cheap and you could also use it whenever you feel the need to purify your body from toxins. As the ingredients are all herbal ones, it would also help you maintain a more nutrient-loaded body.

Using Body Detox For Drug Testing

If you have a drug test which you badly need to pass, a body detox would also help you. By doing the right body detox, you are able to rid your body from any impurities.

However, this only works if your drug test is based on your urine. There are several body detox products for drugs testing but they won't provide your body with any nutrients whatsoever. It will color your urine so that it isn't clear.

Drug detox drinks work by you drinking it and then following up by taking several glasses of water. You need to do this a few hours before you take a drug test. After drinking a few glasses of water, you could easily pass the urine drug test. You would find that your urine is a little yellowish because of the added herbal remedies. Such herbal remedies that are used in drug detox are undetectable by drug tests.

****

Regardless of the reason for detoxification, you need to make sure to only use natural remedies that don't contain any chemicals. Detoxification is a natural process and you should only use natural herbs. It doesn't matter if you use pills, herbs or solution; it is guaranteed that you will feel much better after going through with this detox process.

Using Body Detox For Cleaning Your Colon

Many people who are into this process of detoxifying their body are interested in colon cleansing. From the comfort of your home, you could use body detox remedies to stop constipation and have a healthier colon. The process of colon cleansing is about eliminating those wastes that are in your body and make sure they are clean.

Like common body detoxification remedies, colon cleansing also have the same form like tablets, drinks or tea. You could also get kits for the same purposes. And like all, you would need to take it with water to ensure that you could help the body detox process.

However, there are also resources from the internet. You can find for colon cleansing recipes and products that would assist you with your colon cleanse. The best time for a colon cleanse is when you have plenty of time to rest and take the solutions.

Make sure that you don't have to be working because you may need constant access to a bathroom. After a colon cleanse, you would generally feel lighter and more energetic.

Colon cleansing is also a great way to lose weight. Many colon cleansing solutions are practically the same with weight loss solutions for body detox. Colon cleansing not only flushes waste out from the colon but also provides the body with nutrients to keep the colon healthy, free from toxins.

It is important to have a healthy colon. This is because a lot of diseases can come from the colon and some of them can be very life-threatening. A good way to ensure that your colon is healthy and to maintain an ideal weight is through body detoxification solutions. Ideally, you should get a solution which is mainly created for colon-cleansing.

To find them, you could purchase them from a food store or through the internet. The main thing after taking those solutions is to drink a lot of water. You should also add natural products to help with the colon cleanse and flush out waste from your system.

Antioxidants are very important when it comes to colon cleansing. It will not only boost you with nutrients but would quicken the cleansing process. One of the most popular remedies is to mix pure grape juice with water. You should look for natural grape juice and not those which you buy from the store as they are filled with sugar.

A common supplement that would help with your colon health is resveratrol. It would also improve the health of your digestive system. Derived from the skin of red grapes, the Resveratrol powder can be mixed with water to easily help a colon cleanse.

Regardless of the diet you are on, colon cleansing once in a while is a great way to ensure that your digestive system is in check. It doesn't matter if you make your own or get it from a store, a colon cleanse every two weeks would do a lot of good for your digestive system.

Natural Body Detox Tips

There might be a lot of products in the market for body detox, but you could easily work towards cleansing your body from the comfort of your home without the use of any products from the market.

For starters, you should look to drink purified water. On a single day, you need to drink at least eight glasses of water to maintain your good health.

Most people don't drink enough water and end up gaining a lot of weight and store those toxins in their body, thus gaining weight. Therein lies the power of water, it helps you flush out toxins from your body.

To decide if you are drinking enough water, you can judge this by the color of your urine. Should you be drinking enough water, your urine would be clear.

However, if you urine is dark, it means that you aren't drinking enough water. Commonly put, your urine is more concentrated in the morning but clearer as the day passes by.

There are many people who dislike drinking water because they don't like having to go to the bathroom so frequently. However, it is important that you do so because it is perhaps the most natural form of body detoxification which is natural.

When you keep yourself hydrated, you will notice that you can maintain your weight much easier. You may even lose weight in the long term.

It is also important to eat rightly. When you are in the body cleanse process, you should consume food which are high in vitamins, minerals and low in fat. You should eat at least seven fruits and vegetables a day to help your digestive system and detoxify your colon. Other food to include as well would include, fish, cranberries and vegetables.

All these would assist you by making you healthier and provide your body with the nutrients needed. It is a true fact that you are what you eat.

Not only do you need to start consuming certain food, you would also need to try cut down certain food. This includes fats, fast food, friend food, sodium and processed foods. They all add toxins to your body and only harm your body in the long term.

If you are into organic food, you can choose them as well. Organic food doesn't have toxins and would keep your body clearer from such impurities.

Exercise also plays an important role in body detoxification. Cardiovascular exercises would help you sweat and eliminate stress from your daily life. A great number of people have a lot of stress in their daily life. From work or home, you can easily be stressed from those different situations.

Stress would affect your body and would affect your body detox process. When you exercise, you not only get in shape and burn calories; you would also sweat out all those toxins in your body.

To further help you, supplements can be used as well. In order to naturally cleanse your body, you could also take multivitamins. They would help you get the nutrients you need that you miss from your daily diet.

Although all these tips can help you, the most important thing towards a healthy lifestyle is to ensure that you have good lifestyle habits and avoid unhealthy toxins. Don't smoke, consume drugs or alcohol. They are all bad habits that would be very bad for your health.

Once cleansing your body becomes natural, you would find that it would get easier over time. In the beginning, it may be tough because your body isn't used to it. But once you have gotten used to it, you will feel healthier over time.

Once you get used to the benefits of body detox, you would naturally get used to the body detox habit. This takes time, but it's worth it.

How To Find For The Right Body Detox Product

When searching for body detox products, you would be amazed at the selection of products available. From resources which you can find online to the health stores, they hold a great selection.

However, one thing you want to make sure is the fact that they are made from natural products. This is the most important thing when seeking body detox products.

Among the different type of products for body detox available include:

- Teas
- Patches
- Tablets
- Formulas (Pre-made)
- Powders (Mix With Water)
- Aromatherapy
- Foot Therapy

Without a doubt, all of these could help you with your detox. All of them could be bought online depending on which one is suitable for you. They may work differently, but they are able to achieve the same results.

In this chapter, we would have a rundown on each of the products and how they suit different types of people.

(a) Teas

Teas are not only good for a body detox but also good for your general health as well. When you drink green tea that is filled with antioxidants and vitamins, it would be even better for your body.

You could easily make a cup of tea and make it either hot or cold. You just need to follow the instructions from the package.

Teas are especially ideal for those who prefer drinking liquid and look for a soothing way to cleanse their body from home. They work slowly, unlike solutions. Green tea is also known as a long-term detox solution.

(b) Patches

This solution is similar to when you want to quit smoking. You could also use a patch if you want to cleanse your body. To use this, you simply put the patch onto your skin and the nutrients are easily absorbed into your bloodstream through your skin. It may take longer for it to happen but it is generally more convenient for those who have busy lifestyles and don't have time for a solution.

To purchase body detox patches, you can get them from outlets or simply the internet. Those places that sell body detox supplies would normally sell those patches as well. If you don't have time for the other solutions, this method is ideal for you. You just put them on and you're done.

(c) Tablets

You'll be surprised as to the number of different tablets that you can use for body detox. Such tablets work slower than solutions but are incredibly effective. Some people even take these tablets consistently on a daily basis to ensure that their body is cleansed.

A majority of the tablets for body detox are made from vitamins or other derivatives of herbs. The most commonly used fruit for body detox is Acai Berry. In most places in the world, Acai Berry is available only in juice or powder form. Many people normally make drinks out of it to ensure a smoother digestive system. However, there are tablets which consist primarily of Acai Berry as well.

Such tablets have a great deal of Acai Berry, together with other nutrients from cranberry and lemons. All these are known to help you flush out and cleanse the system effectively.

These tablets are available in most health food stores, local drugstores or online places. The main thing to ensure is that the ingredients in those tablets are all natural.

(d) Formulas (Pre-Made)

Formulas which are pre-made are perhaps the most expensive of all the different kinds of product you can buy. This is because they are already made and can be used as it is. If you are busy, this solution is perhaps the best for you.

You can get such formulas from different outlets from health food stores and through the internet. Using such pre-made formulas is easy. Just follow the instructions and you can perform cleansing from home. There are many different solutions, available in different flavors. They are loaded with multiple vitamins and juices.

Such pre-made formulas are extremely ideal for those who are busy. It is effective and wouldn't take too much time to make. You can also use this with other methods in order to get the best out of a body cleanse.

(e) Powders (Mix With Water)

For fast solutions but a cheaper alternative (than pre-made formulas), powders are perhaps the best for you. With powders, you don't have to pay as much. Besides you could also create your own body detox solutions with the powder that you purchase.

You just need to mix those powders with water and you could just drink them easily. There are many different form of flavors and you can even get a pack of different flavors. You can try several different flavors to decide the one which you like best.

Similarly to pre-made solutions, you mix those powders according to the instructions according to the label. Do remember that different products have different directions and you need to read them carefully.

(f) Aromatherapy

Aromatherapy is another method of cleansing your body which may surprise you. You can use aromatherapy in two ways. First, you can put those essential oils on your skin and allow them to breathe in. Those oils, which are derived from lemon and tea tree leaves would help to cleanse your body.

One important thing to remember when doing so is to not mix those essential oils with carrier oils like canola oil and gently massage them into your skin. Your skin would absorb those essential oils and go into your bloodstream.

Besides that, you could also inhale aromatherapy into your lungs. They also help in transporting these nutrients into your bloodstream. You will however need an infuser to inhale them.

For a long term solution, aromatherapy is good for body detox. It doesn't work immediately, but you cannot doubt its effectiveness. It works like patches as it gets absorbed into your bloodstream and cleans your entire body, including your digestive system.

(g) Foot Therapy

You may be surprised by the power of foot therapy on your digestive system. Your feet are the pathway to your inner body and it would help cleanse your body from toxins. Foot therapy normally includes massage or magnetic therapy.

They are equally effective for the long term. When practicing foot therapy from home, you could use these homemade remedies. It is normally used with other detox methods as well. It could also ensure your long term health. Find for someone who knows about foot therapy and ask them to advice you about it.

You will be amazed by this amazing miracle of massaging your feet to improve your well-being.

Remedies To Drink

From the comfort of your home, you could make homemade remedies which you can drink and help with your body detoxification. In this chapter, I would share the different remedies which you can use and the place to get those body detoxification solutions.

When making these remedies, remember to only use purified water. To get purified water you could head to the grocery store or you could get it from your tap if you have a purifying system in your house.

If you don't have a purifying system in your house, it is great to invest in one. This would help your body clean itself. Water is an essential tool for you're a healthy digestive system. When you drink clean water, your body would be less of toxins.

#1 - Tropical Delight

What You Need:

- Half A Banana
- One Teaspoon Of Flax Seed Oil
- Two Teaspoons Of Pure Lemon Juice
- Ice Cubes Made From Purified Water
- Half A Cup Of Orange Juice
- Quarter Cup Of Acai Juice

Steps:

Put all the ingredients into a blender and mix it. Add the enough ice cubes to ensure that the blender is full.

Drink the whole potion. This drink makes you very full and could be used as a meal as well.

#2 - Colon Cleanse Diet

What You Need:

- One Package Of Green Tea
- One Teaspoon Of Flax Seed Oil
- One Teaspoon Of Fresh Ginger
- One Teaspoon Of Grape Seed Oil
- One Glass Of Water

Steps:

This is a remedy which works well as a colon cleanser.

First thing is to add those ingredients together, and then mix it with the water. To grind the ginger you may need mortar and pestle. However, if you happen to have a food processer, you can use it too. Remember to only use fresh ginger.

Then, open up the green tea package and mix it together. From here, mix everything with water and then drink it.

Gulp down another two glasses of water. Besides, this is also a very good detox remedy if you are looking to lose weight.

#3 - Energizing Cleanse

What You Need:

- One Teaspoon Of Ginseng
- One Teaspoon Of Maca Root
- One Teaspoon Of Acai Powder
- One Glass Of Water

Steps:

To break up the Maca Roots, you may need a pestle and mortar. You need to ensure that they are fresh.

Although it is better to purchase the Ginseng in capsule form, you can also use liquid Ginseng.

Start by grinding the dry ingredients and mix them with the Acai powder; and then with the glass of water.

Drink the mixture and then drink another glass of water to help you get the best out of it.

This remedy wouldn't only give you more energy but would also help detox your digestive system. You could purchase all the ingredients from a health store or even through your online store.

You need to make sure that those ingredients are pure and not chemically produced.

#4 - Vitamin Cleanser

What You Need:

- One Capsule Of Vitamin D, A & K; each
- Half A Teaspoon Of Cinnamon
- One Cup Of Green Tea (Hot)

Steps:

Grind those three capsules into a mortar. Add then into the hot green tea to ensure that they are dissolve.

Add cinnamon into the mixture and slowly drink it down. This mixture adds vitamins and nutrients into your body that you may lack. This is good for stress elimination and is very good for the heart.

All the ingredients could be found from your grocery store. Make sure that you purchase only pure ingredients. The mortar and pestle could be bought online or from other drugstores.

#5 - Cinnamon Spice

What You Need:

- Half A Teaspoon Of Cinnamon
- One Teaspoon Of Honey
- One Cup Of Brewed Green Tea

Steps:

Once you have brewed the green tea, slowly add the cinnamon and honey. Make sure the mixture is still hot and drink it.

It taste very delicious and would cleanse your body and help your heart. It is also very relaxing.

#6 - Lemon Pepper Cleanser

Lemon and pepper, if combined, would help extremely well as a cleanser for your body. This remedy is a very easy but effective cleansing method.

What You Need:

- 2 Teaspoons Of Lemon Zest
- Half A Teaspoon Of Black Pepper
- A Glass Of Water (8 Ounces)

Steps:

Combine all the ingredients and drink it in one go. Once you are done with it, drink about two glasses of water.

The water plays a role of flushing the solution into your digestive system. This remedy is great for your colon and your whole digestive system. You should try to find for fresh ground black pepper and lemon zest.

If you dislike the taste of black pepper, you could remove the black pepper and add a teaspoon of fresh lemon juice.

#7 - Kidney Cleansing

What You Need:

- Three Teaspoons Of Orange Juice
- Half A Cup Of Pure Cranberry Juice
- A Quarter Of A Cup Of Pure Acai Juice
- A Glass Of Water

Steps:

Mix all ingredients together. Add them to the glass of water. Drink it and then drink another two glasses of water.

This remedy would help you clean out your urinary tract and remove infections.

Note: Use only pure ingredients.

#8 - Tropical Detox

What You Need:

- One Banana
- A Cup Of Plain and Unsweetened Yogurt
- Half A Cup Of Pure Orange Juice
- Half A Cup Of Pure Pineapple Juice

Steps:

Insert all ingredients into a blender and mix them well. This is more than a shake, but it is highly effective in cleansing your digestive tract and provides the essential nutrients to your body.

This works slowly, but is extremely healthy for your colon, heart and immune system. Use only fresh ingredients and pure juice.

#9 - Berry Detox

What You Need:

- Half A Cup Of Blueberries
- Four Fresh Strawberries
- Three Quarters Glass Of Water
- A Quarter Glass Of Pure Acai Berry Juice

Steps:

Insert all of those ingredients into a blender and mix them. Drink them immediately.

After that, drink another glass of clean, purified water. This acts as a detoxifier, loaded with antioxidants and purifiers. Remember to only use fresh ingredients.

#10 - Italian Body Detoxifier

What You Need:

- One Teaspoon Of Basil (or Rosemary)
- One Teaspoon Of Oregano
- One Teaspoon Of Flex Seed Oil
- Half A Teaspoon Of Garlic
- A Glass Of Water

Steps:

Combine those ingredients with water and drink it immediately.

Once you are done drinking, wait for another five minutes so that the solution settles. After that, drink two glasses of water without stopping. This is very important as it acts as a detoxifier for your whole body. It helps your digestive and circulatory system.

To get the best results, make sure that those ingredients are fresh.

#11 - Lavender Cleansing

What You Need:

- One Teaspoon Of Flax Seed Oil
- One Teaspoon Of Pure Lavender Oil
- One Glass Of Water

Steps:

Simply mix both oils with water. Drink it.

Take another glass of water to flush down that mixture. This remedy is a full body-cleanse and detoxify you entire digestive system.

#12 - Veggie Cleanser

What You Need:

- One Teaspoon Of Omega Fish Oil
- One Teaspoon Of Flax Seed Oil
- Two Crowns Of Broccoli
- One Peeled Carrot (Fresh)
- Ice Cubes

Steps:

For this recipe, you need a food processor. It would cleans out your system thoroughly and work well on your digestive system.

One thing you need to remember to do is to pulverize vegetables so they are like mush.

From here, add some ice cubes and oils to the mixture. Mix it well.

Drink it. After that, gulp down another glass of clean purified water. This is a drink you could drink regularly. It would even be a substitute for a meal if you want to diet.

Home Made Remedies For Your Skin

To detoxify your body, the best way is by drinking solutions. However, there are other alternative. Some people wouldn't want to drink solutions because of different reasons. They also want body detoxification but find it hard to drink solutions.

If you want to detox your body for the long term, using massage oils from essential oils is one great way. You should never use essential oils directly on your skin, unless you are using Rose and Lavender. As discussed in the previous chapters, aromatherapy works to detox your body in a slower manner.

You could easily find essential oil for these recipes online or from other health stores. Using pure essential oils or extracts for these recipes are very important. Using synthetic ones would not bring the same results as using pure ones. Always remember that.

All these recipes in the next few pages are all safe to use as massage oil.

#1 - Tea Tree Oil & Lemon

When it comes to helping your digestive system, tree tea oil and lemon oil are extremely useful. This is also great for losing weight and clearing out your digestive system. You can easily mix this at home and use it as a form of massage oil or use it in an infuser.

What You Need:

- Half A Teaspoon Of Tea Tree Oil
- Half A Teaspoon Of Pure Lemon Oil
- One Cup Of Carrier Oil (like Canola Oil)

Steps:

Mix all three oils in a brown bottle and shake. The step to using them is the same as with other aromatherapy massage oils. You could also inhale them with an infuser.

It is very important to only get pure lemon oil and not lemon juice. Pure lemon extract can be a substitute for this form of detox, if you couldn't find pure lemon oil.

Tea Tree Oil is something you can find at most health stores. You only need to make sure that they are pure.

#2 - Frankincense

This has been used as a form of healing potent for a few centuries. You can use this remedy to get rid of body toxins and assist with your circulatory system.

What You Need:

- One Teaspoon Of Pure Frankincense
- One Cup Of Carrier Oil (like Canola Oil)

Steps:

Mix both the oils together and put them into a dark bottle with a lid. Once they are mixed, it could be used for massage oil.

Rub the soles of your feet with this oil mixture. Also put the on your chest. It would do wonders from your circulatory system and the scent is very nice. Have a partner to massage your back if you have one.

Canola oil is something that you can get in any grocery store. Frankincense is very common and could be found in almost any health food stores. Like for most recipes, only use the pure form.

With this oil, you can also put them in an infuser to breathe in.

#3 - Lavender and Rose

This is perhaps the easiest of all the aromatherapy detoxification recipes. It would combine two essential oils which are very safe. It wouldn't only relax you, but also cleanse your body of toxins.

What You Need:

- Half A Cup Of Lavender Oil
- Quarter Cup Of Rose Oil

Steps:

Mix both the oil together. You can use it to massage your neck, feet and chest. The oils would be absorbed into your skin and slowly into your blood stream.

If you are tense and want a little relaxation, this is a good mixture.

You could also put the oil into an infuser and breathe the scent. You would be able to absorb the nutrients into your lungs.

You could also put them into your bath and you can soak in it. You will instantly feel relaxed as you would be breathing in oil but also allow those nutrients to soak into your bloodstream from your skin.

Note: Lavender and rose are the safest essential oil to put directly on your skin.

#4 - Almond

This is a recipe that you can use from readily available extracts from the grocery store. When using these extracts, you should still use carrier oil.

What You Need:

- One Teaspoon Of Pure Vanilla Extract
- One Teaspoon Of Pure Almond Extract
- One Cup Of Carrier Oil (like Canola Oil)

Steps:

Combine all three products and shake in a bottle. The mixture can then be applied on your skin.

It has a very nice scent. You could also burn the oils in an infuser. This body detox would help bolster you're your immunity and clean out any toxins.

These ingredients can be found easily from any health store.

With massage therapy and breathing in essential oils is a great way to detox your body from the comfort of your home. Additionally,,, you should practice good lifestyle habits like not taking alcohol and drinking a lot of water.

Staying Detoxified

Body detoxification from the comfort of your home is easy and you have many choices to choose from. There are many different types of remedies which you can use successfully.

When starting, you should start slow. Don't push yourself too much. Start with taking some detox teas. Buy them from a health store and start drinking them on a daily basis.

Going online, you would see that there are many different choices of body detox products. From detox kits, pills, teas and drinks; you would get all of them from the comfort of your home and they will be sent to you.

They all work amazingly in detoxifying your body but they aren't magic cure. Don't abuse your body and then expect to detox time and again. It doesn't work that way. You still need to incorporate healthy habits into your life.

When you perform a home detoxification, you can slowly get rid of toxins from your body and come clean. If you are someone who has been abusing substances and want a change in your lifestyle, you could clean up your body from home and use those body detoxification formulas shared with you in this book.

It is recommended that you use a colon cleanser before starting with a body detox system. This helps you clean your colon and allows your body to be more receptive to the nutrients that you are inserting into your body. The start of a healthy body begins with a healthy digestive tract.

To ensure that you are detoxified, use the body detox system every week for a day and eat a healthier and balanced diet. You also need to make sure that you consume a lot of water and exercise on a regular basis. For some people, vitamins or supplements could also help you be healthier.

Body detox could also help you get in better shape. You need to follow through with the systems and methods share in this book. Don't stop it half way. If you find it tough, try to persevere past it.

Start your detox again to ensure that you have a good health and your body is rid of toxins. Body detoxification is a great way towards maintaining a good health. Start it today!

Resource 1 - Total Wellness Cleanse

This is perhaps the simplest and most powerful natural detox strategy that I have seen. **It has helped more than 19,375 men and women between the ages of 26 and 60.**

This system allows you to:

- Remove Fat
- Fix Life-Threatening Illness
- Give You An Abundance Of Energy Throughout The Day

Check it out at:

http://detoxdiet.wellbeingvalley.com/

Resource 2 - Master Cleansing Secrets

This system is very tough!!!

Before even trying this, make sure that you are ready for it. **Most people can't even last a single day on this system.**

But, I have tried this system and it works miraculously. After trying this system, you would feel:

- Better Appetite
- Feel More Youthful
- Lose Weight In Just A Couple Of Days
- Energy Levels Will Soar

Check it out at:

http://mastercleanse.wellbeingvalley.com/

www.ingramcontent.com/pod-product-compliance
Lightning Source LLC
Chambersburg PA
CBHW070550290526
45790CB00002B/625